Bladder Bliss:
A Guide to Optimal Urinary
Tract Health for Women

PROSSY PRESS

Table of Contents

.Introduction to Urinary Tract Health

A. Understanding the Urinary Tract System

B. Common Urinary Tract Problems for Women

C. The Importance of Good Urinary Tract Health

II. Lifestyle Changes for Optimal Urinary Tract Health

A. Hydration

B. Exercise

C. Dietary Changes

D. Stress Management

III. Natural Supplements and Herbs for Urinary Tract Health

A. Cranberry

B. D-Mannose

C. Uva Ursi

D. Magnesium

E. Vitamin D

IV. Urinary Tract Infections and Prevention

A. Understanding UTIs

B. Risk Factors for UTIs

C. Prevention Techniques

D. Antibiotics and Alternative Treatments

V. Bladder Health and Incontinence

A. Understanding Bladder Health

B. Causes of Incontinence

C. Treatment Options

D. Pelvic Floor Exercises for Improved Bladder Control

VI. Menopause and Urinary Tract Health

A. Understanding Menopause and Its Effects

B. Urinary Tract Changes During Menopause

C. Treatment Options for Menopausal Urinary Tract Issues

VII. Conclusion

Empowering Women to Take Control of Their Urinary Tract Health

I. Introduction to Urinary Tract Health

The urinary system is a critical element of the body that plays a significant function in the disposal of waste and excess fluid from the body. Keeping the urinary tract healthy is vital for general well-being, since abnormalities in this system may lead to a variety of unpleasant and even painful symptoms.

The urinary system is made up of the kidneys, ureters, bladder, and urethra. The kidneys are two bean-shaped organs placed in the lower back, right above the waist. Their major purpose is to filter waste and excess fluid from the blood, which is subsequently removed from the body as urine. The ureters are small tubes that link the kidneys to the bladder, enabling the urine to move from the kidneys to the bladder.

The bladder is a muscle sac found in the pelvis that retains urine until it is removed from the body. The urethra is a small tube that transfers urine from the bladder to the exterior of the body. The length of the urethra varies between men and women, with males having a longer urethra that extends through the penis and women having a shorter urethra that opens in front of the vagina.

Maintaining excellent urinary system health is vital for avoiding the development of uncomfortable and possibly dangerous illnesses, such as urinary tract infections (UTIs), bladder stones, and interstitial cystitis. UTIs are bacterial infections that develop in the urinary system and are one of the most prevalent forms of illnesses. Symptoms of UTIs include painful urination, frequent urination, and murky or strong-smelling urine. Bladder stones are hard lumps that develop in the bladder and may cause pain and trouble urinating. Interstitial cystitis is a disorder that causes bladder discomfort and frequent urination, although the reason is not entirely known.

Fortunately, there are several actions that you may do to promote the health of your urinary tract. One of the most essential things is to keep hydrated by drinking enough water throughout the day. This helps flush out germs and waste materials, minimizing the risk of UTIs and other illnesses.

It is also crucial to exercise basic hygiene, particularly after using the restroom. This involves wiping from front to back to prevent germs from migrating from the anus to the urethra. Women should also avoid using irritating feminine hygiene products, such as douches and powders, since they may irritate the urinary tract and increase the risk of infections.

Another strategy to maintain the health of your urinary tract is to frequently participate in physical exercise, since this may assist improve bladder control and minimize the risk of UTIs. Kegel exercises, which include contracting and releasing the pelvic floor muscles, are particularly effective for improving bladder control.

It is also vital to maintain a healthy diet, since some foods might impact the health of the urinary system. For example, meals and beverages that are heavy in sugar and caffeine may irritate the bladder and increase the risk of UTIs. On the other hand, eating a diet that is high in fiber and contains lots of fruits and vegetables may assist promote the health of the urinary system.

In addition to adopting lifestyle changes, it is crucial to seek medical assistance if you encounter any symptoms that signal a problem with your urinary system. This involves painful urination, frequent urination, and hazy or strong-smelling urine. Your doctor may identify the underlying issue and propose a suitable treatment approach.

In conclusion, the urinary system is a key portion of the body that plays a significant function in the disposal of waste and excess fluid. Keeping the urinary system healthy is vital for general well-being, and there are several actions that you can take to promote its health. By remaining hydrated, maintaining proper hygiene, and participating in physical activity .

A. Understanding the Urinary Tract System

The urinary tract system is a sophisticated and complicated network of organs that work together to eliminate waste from the body and maintain the body's fluid balance. This system comprises multiple organs, including the kidneys, ureters, bladder, and urethra. Understanding the urinary tract system is vital for maintaining general health and avoiding problems such as urinary tract infections, kidney disease, and bladder control concerns.

The kidneys are the principal component of the urinary tract system and are responsible for filtering waste and excess fluid from the circulation. They are positioned in the upper belly and are shaped like beans. The kidneys collect blood from the renal arteries and filter it via small filters called nephrons. The waste and excess fluid are removed from the circulation and are delivered to the ureters, which are thin tubes that link the kidneys to the bladder.

The bladder is a sac-like structure found in the lower abdomen and is responsible for retaining pee. When the bladder is full, it sends signals to the brain suggesting the urge to pee. The muscles in the bladder then contract to evacuate the pee into the urethra. The urethra is a thin tube that transports urine from the bladder out of the body.

The urinary tract system is crucial for eliminating waste from the body and maintaining fluid equilibrium. The kidneys are responsible for filtering waste and excess fluid from the blood and eliminating it from the body via the ureters, bladder, and urethra. The bladder stores urine until it is time to pee and the urethra delivers the urine out of the body.

One of the most prevalent disorders with the urinary tract system is a urinary tract infection (UTI) (UTI). UTIs are infections that develop in the urinary system and are typically caused by bacteria. Symptoms of a UTI include painful urination, frequent desires to pee, and murky or strong-smelling urine. UTIs may be treated with medication and can be avoided by keeping hydrated, wiping front to back after using the toilet, and avoiding bubble baths and tight-fitting clothes.

Another prevalent concern with the urinary tract system is kidney disease. Kidney disease is a disorder in which the kidneys are damaged and unable to filter waste from the blood. Symptoms of kidney illness include weariness, swelling in the legs and ankles, and changes in urine production. Kidney disease may be managed with medicine and lifestyle adjustments, such as a low-sodium diet and frequent exercise.

Bladder control difficulties, commonly known as urine incontinence, are another issue that may develop with the urinary tract system. Urinary incontinence is the loss of bladder control and may be caused by a number of causes, including pregnancy, aging, and nerve injury. Symptoms of urinary incontinence include leaks, unexpected desires to pee, and problems retaining urine. Treatment for urine incontinence may involve pelvic floor exercises, medication, and in extreme situations, surgery.

Generally, knowing the urinary tract system is vital for maintaining overall health and avoiding problems such as UTIs, kidney disease, and bladder control concerns. Regular check-ups with a healthcare practitioner may help identify and prevent issues before they become severe. It is also crucial to keep hydrated, exercise proper hygiene, and adopt lifestyle modifications to promote the health of the urinary tract system.

In conclusion, the urinary tract system is a complicated network of organs that work together to eliminate waste from the body and maintain fluid equilibrium. Understanding this system is vital for maintaining general health and avoiding problems such as UTIs, renal disease, and bladder control concerns. Regular check-ups and keeping a healthy lifestyle may assist promote the health of the urinary tract system and prevent issues from arising.

Urinary tract difficulties are frequent in women of all ages and may be caused by a range of reasons such as infection, injury, and underlying medical diseases. These disorders may vary from minor to severe and can cause discomfort, agony, and even life-threatening illnesses if not addressed swiftly. Understanding the most prevalent urinary tract disorders for women and their symptoms, causes, and therapies is vital for ensuring quick and efficient therapy.

Urinary Tract Infection (UTI) (UTI)

UTIs are one of the most frequent urinary tract diseases in women. They are caused by bacteria that enter the urethra and grow in the bladder, producing irritation and infection. Women are more prone to UTIs than males owing to their anatomy, with the female urethra being shorter than the male urethra, making it easier for germs to enter the bladder. Common symptoms of UTIs include discomfort or burning during urination, frequent urination, murky or bloody urine, and lower abdomen ache.

UTIs may be treated with antibiotics given by a doctor. It is crucial to finish the whole course of antibiotics even if symptoms have improved. It is also crucial to drink enough water to wash out the germs and avoid dehydration.

Interstitial Cystitis (IC) (IC)

Interstitial cystitis is a persistent illness that produces discomfort or pressure in the bladder and pelvic area. The etiology of IC is unclear, although it is thought to be associated with a flaw in the bladder lining that enables toxic chemicals to infiltrate and irritate the bladder wall. Common symptoms of IC include frequent urination, discomfort during urination, and pain in the pelvic area.

Treatment for IC might include drugs to relieve discomfort and inflammation, bladder instillations, and lifestyle adjustments such as avoiding bladder irritants like coffee and alcohol. In extreme circumstances, surgery may be indicated.

Overactive Bladder (OAB) (OAB)

Overactive bladder is a disorder when the muscles of the bladder spasm suddenly, prompting an urgent desire to pee. It is a typical concern for women, particularly after menopause. Common symptoms of OAB include frequent urination, urgent need to pee, and waking up at night to urinate.

Treatment for OAB might include drugs to relax the bladder muscles, bladder retraining, and lifestyle modifications such as lowering fluid consumption before night. In extreme circumstances, surgery may be indicated.

Stress Urinary Incontinence (SUI) (SUI)

Stress urinary incontinence is a disorder where women have leakage of pee during actions that increase strain on the bladder, such as coughing, sneezing, or exercising. It is a prevalent condition in women following pregnancy, delivery, and menopause. Common symptoms of SUI include leaking of urine during activities that increase strain on the bladder, trouble regulating urination, and waking up at night to pee.

Treatment for SUI might involve pelvic floor exercises, bladder retraining, and lifestyle modifications such as lowering fluid consumption before night. In extreme circumstances, surgery may be indicated.

Vesicovaginal Fistula (VVF) (VVF)

Vesicovaginal fistula is a condition where a link develops between the bladder and the vagina, allowing urine to seep into the vagina. It is an uncommon disorder that may emerge after delivery, injury, or surgery. Common symptoms of VVF include leaking of urine into the vagina, frequent urination, and pain during sexual intercourse.

Treatment for VVF might involve surgery to restore the link between the bladder and vagina. In certain circumstances, the fistula may heal on its own with adequate care.

C. The Importance of Good Urinary Tract Health

Urinary tract health is vital for general health and well-being. The urinary tract is a complicated system responsible for filtering and removing waste and surplus fluids from the body. Good urinary tract health is vital to avoid infections, preserve kidney function, and guarantee the appropriate functioning of other organs. In this post, we'll examine the necessity of having a healthy urinary tract and how to attain it.

The urinary system is made up of various elements, including the kidneys, ureters, bladder, and urethra. The kidneys are responsible for filtering waste and surplus fluids from the circulation and creating urine. The ureters transport urine from the kidneys to the bladder, where it is kept until it's evacuated via the urethra. Good urinary tract health is crucial to guarantee the appropriate functioning of each of these elements.

One of the key reasons why excellent urinary tract health is crucial is to avoid infections. The urinary system is sensitive to infections, particularly in women. Women have a shorter urethra than males, which makes it simpler for germs to enter the bladder and create an infection. Symptoms of a urinary tract infection include frequent urination, discomfort or burning during urination, murky or strong-smelling urine, and pressure in the lower abdomen. If left untreated, a urinary tract infection may move to the kidneys and cause major health complications.

In addition to avoiding infections, proper urinary tract health is necessary to preserve kidney function. The kidneys perform a key function in filtering waste and excess fluids from the circulation. If the urinary system is not operating correctly, the kidneys may get damaged and lose their capacity to filter waste. This may lead to major health complications, such as renal failure and excessive blood pressure.

Good urinary tract health is also crucial for the correct functioning of other organs. The bladder and urethra play a key function in regulating the discharge of urine. If the urinary system is not operating correctly, it may induce incontinence, which can be a source of shame and suffering. In addition, the bladder and urethra serve to maintain adequate pressure in the pelvis, which is vital for sexual and reproductive health.

So, how can you keep your urinary tract healthy? Here are some tips:

Drink lots of water: Staying hydrated is vital to avoid infections and maintain good kidney function. Aim to drink at least eight glasses of water every day.

Avoid irritants: Certain meals and beverages might irritate the urinary system and increase the risk of infection. Examples include alcohol, coffee, and spicy meals.

Wipe front to back: This helps to avoid the transmission of germs from the anus to the urethra, which may raise the risk of infection.

Empty your bladder regularly: Holding urine in the bladder for lengthy periods of time might raise the risk of infection. Try to empty your bladder every three to four hours.

Wear breathable underwear: Wearing tight-fitting underwear or trousers may trap moisture and increase the risk of infection. Choose underwear made from breathable fabrics, such as cotton.

Practice excellent hygiene: Regular cleaning of the genital region might assist to avoid infections. It's also crucial to change out of damp gear, such as swimwear or gym clothes, as soon as possible.

In conclusion, maintaining healthy urinary tract health is vital for general health and well-being. By following the advice presented in this article, you may assist to avoid infections, preserve kidney function, and guarantee the normal functioning of other organs. If you have signs of a urinary tract infection or any other health concerns, get medical assistance as soon as possible.

II. Lifestyle Changes for Optimal Urinary Tract Health

A. Hydration

Hydration is a key element of maintaining a healthy lifestyle, and it plays a critical role in maintaining good urinary tract health. Your body requires a steady supply of water to operate correctly, and this is particularly true for your urinary system. Staying hydrated helps to flush out waste materials, avoid urinary tract infections (UTIs), and preserve bladder health.

The urinary tract is responsible for filtering waste from your bloodstream and excreting it from your body. This procedure includes a range of organs, including the kidneys, ureters, bladder, and urethra. The kidneys are responsible for filtering waste materials and maintaining your body's fluid levels, while the ureters transport urine from the kidneys to the bladder. The bladder retains urine until it is removed from the body via the urethra.

One of the major methods to maintain good urinary tract health is to keep hydrated. Adequate hydration helps to avoid UTIs, which may be unpleasant and cause discomfort. UTIs are caused by bacteria that enter the urinary system and grow, causing irritation and infection. Hydration helps to wash away germs from the urinary system, lowering the incidence of UTIs.

Drinking adequate water also helps to preserve bladder health. The bladder is a muscle that has to be maintained strong to operate effectively. If you are dehydrated, your bladder may become weaker, which can lead to incontinence, frequent visits to the toilet, and other urinary issues. Staying hydrated helps to keep your bladder robust and operating correctly.

Another advantage of being hydrated is that it may assist to lower the chance of kidney stones. Kidney stones are created when waste items in the urine get concentrated and form solid masses. Drinking adequate water helps to dilute the urine, minimizing the chance of kidney stones developing.

In addition to water, there are additional liquids that may assist to maintain excellent urinary tract health. Cranberry juice, for example, is commonly suggested to help avoid UTIs. Cranberries contain chemicals that inhibit germs from sticking to the urinary system, lowering the risk of infection.

It is vital to know that not all beverages are helpful for your urinary system. Caffeinated beverages, such as coffee and tea, may dehydrate the body, making it more difficult to maintain ideal urinary tract health. Alcoholic drinks may also be troublesome, since they can irritate the bladder and increase the risk of UTIs.

So how much water should you be drinking each day to ensure optimum urinary tract health? The quantity of water you require depends on a variety of variables, including your age, weight, and activity level. A common advice is to drink at least eight glasses of water each day. This might be in the form of water, tea, juice, or other non-caffeinated liquids.

It is also crucial to pay attention to your body's thirst signals. If you are feeling thirsty, it is an indication that you need to drink more water. You may also check your urine color to detect whether you are dehydrated. If your pee is light yellow, it implies you are well hydrated. If it is dark yellow or amber, it is a warning that you need to drink more water.

In conclusion, hydration is a key part of maintaining healthy urinary tract health. Drinking adequate water helps to flush out waste materials, avoid UTIs, and preserve bladder health. It is crucial to drink at least eight glasses of water each day, and to pay heed to your body's thirst signals. By making water a priority, you may assist to maintain a healthy urinary system and avoid urinary issues.

B. Exercise

Exercise has been demonstrated to be one of the most beneficial lifestyle improvements for good urinary tract health. Regular exercise not only boosts general physical health but also delivers several advantages to the urinary system. In this post, we will discuss the numerous ways in which exercise may promote urinary tract health, and how it can be included into your daily routine.

One of the most important advantages of exercise for urinary tract health is its capacity to promote bladder control. Exercise strengthens the muscles in the pelvic area, especially the muscles involved for bladder control. Regular exercise, such as pelvic floor muscle exercises, can help to improve bladder control and prevent incontinence, a common problem among women and older individuals.

In addition, exercise may assist to enhance bladder function by improving the flow of urine and avoiding urinary retention. Regular exercise promotes blood flow and oxygenation to the urinary system, which helps to flush out dangerous germs and prevent urinary tract infections (UTIs) (UTIs). Furthermore, exercise helps to avoid constipation, which may also lead to UTIs, by encouraging regular bowel movements.

Exercise may also help to decrease stress, which is a major cause for UTIs. When we are under stress, our body creates stress chemicals that may impair our immune system and raise the risk of infections. Exercise has been demonstrated to lower stress and boost the immune system, decreasing the incidence of UTIs and other urinary tract issues.

Another advantage of exercise for urinary tract health is its capacity to enhance sleep. Good sleep is critical for general health, and it is also important for urinary tract health. When we sleep, our body is able to flush away dangerous germs from the urinary system, avoiding UTIs and other illnesses. Exercise helps to promote sleep by lowering stress, calming the body, and encouraging physical relaxation.

Exercise may also assist to maintain a healthy weight, which is vital for urinary tract health. Being overweight or obese may place additional strain on the bladder and lead to incontinence, UTIs, and other urinary system disorders. Regular exercise, along with a good diet, may assist to maintain a healthy weight and avoid these disorders.

Finally, exercise may assist to promote mental health and well-being, which is also crucial for urinary tract health. Exercise has been demonstrated to increase mood, decrease stress, and avoid depression and anxiety. These advantages may minimize the risk of UTIs and other urinary tract issues, and enhance overall quality of life.

Incorporating fitness into your everyday routine is simpler than you would believe. The ideal kind of exercise for urinary tract health is low-impact exercises, such as walking, swimming, or cycling. These exercises serve to strengthen the muscles in the pelvic area, enhance blood flow, and improve bladder function, without placing too much stress on the bladder or urinary system.

It is advised that you strive for 30 minutes of moderate-intensity exercise, such as brisk walking, five times a week. If you are new to exercise, start with 10-15 minutes of exercise a day and gradually increase the amount of time you spend exercising as your fitness improves. You may also add exercise into your everyday routine by taking the stairs instead of the elevator, walking instead of driving, or taking a break from sitting to stretch and move your body.

In conclusion, exercise is one of the most beneficial lifestyle adjustments for excellent urinary tract health. Regular exercise may enhance bladder control, bladder function, decrease stress, improve sleep, maintain a healthy weight, and promote mental health and well-being. Incorporating exercise into your regular routine is straightforward, and the advantages are many. So, what are you waiting for? Get active now and experience a healthy urinary tract!

C. Dietary Changes

Dietary Changes for Optimal Urinary Tract Health

The urinary system is a critical component of our body, responsible for filtering and excreting waste items from our bloodstream. To maintain good urinary tract health, it is vital to include numerous lifestyle adjustments, including dietary changes. In this post, we will look into the many dietary modifications that one may undertake to guarantee a healthy urinary system.

Hydration: Hydration is of vital significance when it comes to keeping a healthy urinary system. The urinary system depends on enough hydration to filter away germs, minerals, and other waste materials. Aim to drink at least 8 glasses of water every day and restrict the use of diuretics such as coffee, tea, and alcohol.

Fiber-rich foods: Fiber is vital in maintaining healthy urinary tract health. It aids in reducing constipation, which is a significant cause of urinary tract infections.

Opt for fiber-rich foods including fruits, vegetables, whole grains, and legumes.

Low-fat foods: A low-fat diet may greatly lower the incidence of urinary tract infections. The high-fat content in some diets stimulates the production of cytokines, which may result in inflammation. To lower the risk of urinary tract infections, it is suggested to limit the intake of animal-based goods such cheese, pork, and butter, and opt for low-fat dairy products and plant-based substitutes.

Acidic foods: Certain acidic meals including citrus fruits, tomatoes, and vinegar may irritate the urinary system, leading to bladder and kidney infections. If you are prone to urinary tract infections, it is advisable to decrease the intake of certain foods.

Bladder irritants: Certain foods may function as bladder irritants, leading to an increase in urine frequency and urgency. These include spicy meals, alcohol, caffeine, and artificial sweeteners. If you are having these symptoms, it is advisable to exclude these items from your diet and see if it makes a difference.

Cranberries: Cranberries are regarded to be useful for urinary tract health since they contain proanthocyanidins, which inhibit germs from attaching to the bladder membrane. The use of cranberry juice or supplements may considerably lower the incidence of urinary tract infections.

Vitamin C: Vitamin C has antimicrobial characteristics and is considered to enhance the immune system, making it a crucial vitamin for good urinary tract health. Opt for foods high in vitamin C, such as citrus fruits, strawberries, kiwi, and bell peppers.

Probiotics: Probiotics are good microorganisms that may aid in keeping a healthy urinary system. They aid in avoiding the formation of dangerous bacteria, which may lead to urinary tract infections. Probiotics may be found in fermented foods like yogurt, kefir, and kombucha, or in supplement form.

In conclusion, dietary adjustments are an important component of maintaining good urinary tract health. It is crucial to maintain hydration, take a diet high in fiber and low in fat, minimize acidic and bladder irritating meals, and integrate foods that are healthy for the urinary system, such as cranberries and probiotics. It is also advisable to seek medical treatment if you are having any signs of a urinary tract infection. By embracing these dietary modifications, you may dramatically minimize the incidence of urinary tract infections and maintain a healthy urinary tract.

D. Stress Management

Stress is a prevalent issue in contemporary life and may impact one's physical and mental health. It has been identified to be a risk factor for a variety of health disorders, including urinary tract infections (UTIs) (UTIs). This is because stress may trigger changes in the body that can contribute to an increased risk of UTIs.

For this reason, stress management is regarded to be one of the lifestyle adjustments that might assist maintain good urinary tract health.

One of the ways in which stress affects the urinary system is by creating alterations in the urinary tract flora. This may result in an excess of dangerous bacteria and an imbalance of the healthy bacteria that typically assist to avoid UTIs. This may make it simpler for UTIs to develop. Additionally, stress may trigger changes in the immune system that might make it more difficult for the body to fight against diseases. This, in turn, raises the risk of UTIs.

To manage stress and support good urinary tract health, there are a variety of lifestyle modifications that may be performed. One of the most effective is exercise. Regular exercise has been found to provide a range of advantages for stress management, including lowering levels of stress hormones, boosting mood, and reducing anxiety and despair. Exercise may also assist to boost the immune system, which can minimize the incidence of UTIs.

Another crucial lifestyle modification is to keep a healthy diet. A nutritious diet may assist to support a healthy urinary system by supplying the body with the nutrients it needs to perform efficiently. Foods that are strong in antioxidants, such as fruits and vegetables, may help to decrease inflammation and enhance the health of the urinary system. Additionally, foods that are rich in fiber may help to prevent UTIs by increasing regular bowel movements and minimizing the amount of time bacteria can thrive in the stomach.

Stress management practices may also be useful in lowering the incidence of UTIs. For example, mindfulness meditation, deep breathing, and yoga have been proved to be useful for lowering stress and increasing general health. These approaches may assist to quiet the mind and minimize emotions of tension and worry. Additionally, they may assist to boost the immune system, which can minimize the incidence of UTIs.

Another helpful strategy to handle stress is to get adequate sleep. Sleep is vital for stress management since it helps to lower levels of stress hormones, enhance mood, and reduce anxiety and despair. Additionally, sleep is vital for the functioning of the immune system, which may assist to lower the incidence of UTIs.

Finally, it is crucial to be cognizant of the influence that stress may have on the urinary tract. If you are suffering symptoms of a UTI, it is crucial to get medical care as soon as possible. This will help to prevent the infection from getting more severe and will also help to lower the chance of consequences.

In conclusion, stress management is a crucial element of supporting good urinary tract health. By making changes to your lifestyle, such as exercising regularly, maintaining a healthy diet, practicing stress management techniques, getting enough sleep, and being mindful of the impact that stress can have on the urinary tract, you can help to reduce your risk of UTIs and promote overall health and well-being.

III. Natural Supplements and Herbs for Urinary Tract Health

A. Cranberry

Cranberry is a tiny, red fruit that is native to North America and has been utilized for ages by indigenous peoples for its health benefits. In recent years, it has gained appeal as a natural supplement and herb for urinary tract health owing to its ability to prevent and cure urinary tract infections (UTIs) (UTIs).

A UTI is an infection that arises in any region of the urinary system, including the bladder, urethra, ureters, and kidneys. UTIs are most usually caused by bacteria and may result in symptoms such as discomfort or burning during urination, frequent urination, and murky or strong-smelling urine.

Cranberry has been reported to be useful in preventing and treating UTIs because of its unique ingredients, including proanthocyanidins, anthocyanins, and organic acids. These substances have been found to inhibit bacteria from sticking to the urinary tract walls, which may help prevent UTIs from forming or reoccurring.

Additionally, cranberries contain antibacterial capabilities that may assist to eradicate dangerous microorganisms in the urinary system. It is also rich in antioxidants and vitamins, especially vitamin C, which may help to improve the immune system and protect against UTIs and other infections.

The usefulness of cranberries for UTI prevention and treatment has been proven by multiple research. One research indicated that women who took cranberry supplements had a considerably decreased incidence of UTIs compared to those who did not take supplements. Another research indicated that consuming cranberry supplements decreased the occurrence of UTIs in women with a history of recurrent UTIs.

It is vital to know that not all cranberry products are made equal. Some cranberry pills have additional sugars or artificial sweeteners, which may be damaging to your health. It is preferable to use a pure, unsweetened cranberry supplement or to consume fresh or dried cranberries as part of a balanced diet.

When using cranberry for UTI prevention or treatment, it is vital to follow the prescribed dose on the product label. Taking too much cranberry may lead to digestive adverse effects, such as nausea and diarrhea
It is also crucial to note that cranberry should not be used as a replacement for antibiotics or other medical therapies for UTIs. If you feel that you have a UTI, it is crucial to consult a doctor for a clear diagnosis and treatment plan.

In conclusion, cranberry is a natural vitamin and plant that has been proved to be useful in preventing and treating urinary tract infections. Its unique components and antioxidant capabilities make it a safe and natural solution for people wishing to boost their urinary tract health. However, it is vital to pick a pure, unsweetened cranberry product and to follow the specified dose to prevent any negative effects. If you feel that you have a UTI, it is crucial to consult a doctor for correct diagnosis and treatment.

B. D-Mannose

D-Mannose is a naturally occurring sugar that is gaining appeal as a supplement for preserving urinary tract health. This sugar may be found in tiny levels in various fruits and vegetables, but is also available in a concentrated form as a nutritional supplement.

Urinary tract infections (UTIs) are a frequent condition that affects many individuals, particularly women. UTIs are caused by bacteria that enter the urinary system and grow, producing symptoms such as pain or discomfort during urination, frequent desires to pee, and murky or strong-smelling urine.

Antibiotics are frequently the first line of therapy for UTIs, but they may have negative effects and can potentially contribute to the growth of antibiotic-resistant bacteria. In recent years, natural medicines such as D-Mannose have emerged as a viable alternative to orthodox treatments.

D-Mannose acts by preventing germs from sticking to the walls of the urinary system. When bacteria enter the urinary system, they cling to the walls and grow, creating an infection. D-Mannose interferes with this attachment mechanism, leading the bacteria to be removed from the body via urine.

Studies have revealed that D-Mannose may be useful in preventing and treating UTIs. In one research, women who took D-Mannose daily for six months had a considerable decrease in the frequency of UTIs they had. Another research indicated that D-Mannose was equally effective as an antibiotic in treating UTIs in women.

D-Mannose is also a safe and well-tolerated supplement. It is taken into the circulation at a modest rate, which implies that it does not have a substantial influence on blood sugar levels. It is also removed from the body via urine, thus it does not accumulate in the body like certain other sugars.

In addition to its advantages for urinary tract health, D-Mannose has also been proven to offer potential benefits for general health. It has been proven to have antioxidant and anti-inflammatory qualities, and may have a good influence on gut health by helping to maintain a healthy balance of bacteria in the stomach.

Despite its rising popularity, D-Mannose is not a cure for UTIs, and it is crucial to seek medical care if you feel that you have an infection. However, taking D-Mannose as a supplement may be a safe and effective strategy to maintain urinary tract health and lower the incidence of UTIs.

If you are contemplating taking D-Mannose, it is vital to consult your healthcare professional first to check that it is safe for you. It is also vital to buy a high-quality supplement that has been verified for purity and efficacy, and to follow the suggested dose.

In conclusion, D-Mannose is a potential natural supplement for sustaining urinary tract health. With its capacity to prevent bacteria from sticking to the walls of the urinary tract, its safety profile, and its potential advantages for general health, it is a good alternative for anybody searching for a natural approach for UTI prevention and treatment.

C. Uva Ursi

Uva Ursi, also known as Bearberry, is a shrub that grows in the Northern Hemisphere and is often used as a natural supplement and herb for urinary tract health. The leaves of this plant contain a chemical called arbutin, which is transformed into hydroquinone in the body and works as an antibacterial agent. This makes Uva Ursi a strong natural medicine for many urinary tract diseases, including cystitis, urethritis, and pyelonephritis.

Urinary tract infections are a prevalent health condition, especially for women. These infections may cause painful urination, frequent urine, and an urgent desire to pee, making it a tough disease to live with. In extreme situations, it may even lead to more major issues such as kidney infections, making it vital to seek quick treatment.

Uva Ursi is often used as a natural cure for urinary tract infections, since it has been proved to help lessen the symptoms and improve general health. It is commonly taken in conjunction with other natural treatments, such as cranberry and dandelion, to boost its potency and give additional health advantages.

One of the key advantages of Uva Ursi is its capacity to suppress the formation of dangerous germs in the urinary system. The hydroquinone generated from arbutin in Uva Ursi functions as an antibacterial agent, eliminating dangerous bacteria and lowering the incidence of urinary tract infections. This natural herb has also been demonstrated to help decrease inflammation and improve general urinary tract health, making it a popular option for individuals trying to enhance their health organically.

In addition to its antibacterial qualities, Uva Ursi also possesses diuretic characteristics. This implies that it helps enhance urine flow, clearing out toxins and dangerous germs from the urinary system. This is especially important for persons with urinary tract infections, as it helps minimize the chance of recurrence and ensures that the urinary system is maintained healthy and operating effectively.

Uva Ursi is also recognized for its astringent characteristics. Astringents force tissues to constrict, lowering swelling and inflammation. This makes it a useful natural cure for lowering the symptoms of urinary tract infections, such as discomfort and burning during urination. It also helps prevent the chance of additional issues, such as bladder infections, by keeping the urinary system healthy and operating appropriately.

Uva Ursi is a safe and natural alternative to over-the-counter medicine for urinary tract health. Unlike other pharmaceuticals, it does not create negative effects or interact with other prescriptions, making it a perfect solution for persons with other health concerns or using other medications.

However, it is vital to note that Uva Ursi should only be taken in moderation. Long-term usage of Uva Ursi may induce liver damage and lead to other health concerns. It is advised that users restrict their usage of Uva Ursi to no more than four weeks at a time, and that they talk with their healthcare physician before beginning any new supplement regimen.

In conclusion, Uva Ursi is a potent natural therapy for urinary tract health. Its antibacterial, diuretic, and astringent characteristics make it a good option for people trying to enhance their health organically. It is a safe and effective alternative to over-the-counter medicine, but it should only be taken in moderation and under the advice of a healthcare expert. If you are suffering symptoms of a urinary tract infection, it is important that you consult with your healthcare practitioner to identify the best course of action for your unique requirements.

D. Magnesium

Magnesium is a naturally occurring mineral that offers various health advantages, including its capacity to enhance urinary tract health. This mineral is vital for numerous activities in the body, including the normal functioning of the muscles, the control of heart rate and blood pressure, and the creation of energy. It is also vital for the health of the bones and teeth. In addition to these advantages, magnesium has been proved to have a favorable influence on urinary tract health, making it a popular option for individuals searching for natural supplements and herbs to boost their general well-being.

The urinary system is a crucial element of the body, responsible for eliminating waste and extra fluid from the body. It is made of the kidneys, ureters, bladder, and urethra. When the urinary system is healthy, it performs easily and efficiently, but when there is a problem, it may produce a variety of symptoms, including pain, discomfort, and infections.

Magnesium has a crucial function in supporting the health of the urinary system. This mineral helps to control the muscular tone in the bladder, limiting involuntary spasms and minimizing the risk of urine incontinence. It also helps to minimize the incidence of urinary tract infections by increasing the formation of good bacteria in the bladder and urethra. This may assist to avoid the proliferation of dangerous bacteria, which can cause illnesses.

In addition, magnesium has been demonstrated to have a favorable influence on bladder health. This mineral helps to relax the muscles of the bladder, lowering the frequency and urgency of urinating. This may be particularly advantageous for patients who have bladder disorders, such as overactive bladder syndrome or interstitial cystitis. By lowering the symptoms of these illnesses, magnesium may assist to enhance overall urinary tract health and quality of life.

Magnesium supplements and herbs are an excellent method to enhance your consumption of this crucial mineral. There are several various types of magnesium available, including magnesium citrate, magnesium glycinate, and magnesium oxide. Some of the greatest natural sources of magnesium are leafy green vegetables, nuts and seeds, and whole grains.

One of the most popular herbs for promoting urinary tract health is cranberry. This plant includes chemicals that serve to inhibit the attachment of dangerous germs to the bladder and urethra, minimizing the incidence of infections. Cranberry also helps to increase the formation of beneficial bacteria in the urinary system, which may assist to avoid the proliferation of dangerous bacteria.

Another prominent herb for urinary tract wellness is uva ursi. This plant contains antibacterial characteristics, which may assist to inhibit the formation of dangerous germs in the urinary system. It is also a natural diuretic, which may assist to flush out toxic toxins and waste from the body, lowering the risk of infections.

In addition to magnesium and herbs, there are numerous additional natural vitamins and therapies that may assist to support urinary tract health. These include probiotics, which may help to improve the balance of bacteria in the urinary system, and vitamin C, which has been demonstrated to help prevent urinary tract infections.

It is crucial to note that although magnesium and other natural supplements and herbs might be good for improving urinary tract health, they should not be used as a replacement for professional medical treatment. If you suffer signs of a urinary tract issue, such as pain or discomfort during urination, frequent or urgent urination, or a persistent need to pee, you should consult a healthcare practitioner for a correct diagnosis and treatment.

In conclusion, magnesium is an essential element for the health of the urinary system, as well as for general well-being. This mineral serves to control the muscular tone in the bladder, minimizing the risk of urine incontinence and bladder issues, and encourages the formation of good bacteria in the urinary system .

E. Vitamin D

Vitamin D is a fat-soluble vitamin that is needed for numerous body activities, including bone health, immune system function, and calcium absorption. It is also known to have a favorable impact on the urinary system and may help avoid urinary tract infections (UTIs) (UTIs). In this post, we will study the advantages of Vitamin D for urinary tract health and why it is regarded as a natural supplement and herb for UTI prevention.

The urinary tract is a complicated system of organs that helps filter waste and surplus fluids from the body. UTIs are a frequent disease for many individuals and are mainly caused by bacteria that enter the urinary system. These infections may produce symptoms such as painful urination, frequent urination, and murky urine. If left untreated, UTIs may lead to more significant health concerns, such as kidney damage.

Vitamin D is known to help prevent UTIs by strengthening the immune system and helping the body fight off dangerous germs. The body creates Vitamin D when the skin is exposed to sunshine, and it may also be received through specific foods, such as fatty fish, dairy products, and eggs. Some studies have indicated that those with low amounts of Vitamin D are more prone to acquire UTIs than those with normal levels.

In addition to its immune-boosting characteristics, Vitamin D also helps control the development and replication of cells in the urinary system. This may help limit the formation of dangerous germs and lower the incidence of UTIs. Additionally, Vitamin D helps the body absorb calcium, which is vital for keeping healthy bones and avoiding osteoporosis. Calcium is also crucial for urinary system health, since it helps the urinary tract muscles work correctly and inhibits the creation of urinary stones.

Vitamin D pills are readily accessible and are commonly advised for those who do not acquire enough Vitamin D via their diet or solar exposure. It is crucial to consult your doctor before taking any new supplement, since they might mix with certain drugs and produce negative effects in some individuals. It is also crucial to have your Vitamin D levels evaluated before taking a supplement, since taking too much Vitamin D may be dangerous.

In conclusion, Vitamin D is a natural vitamin and herb that may help prevent UTIs and improve overall urinary tract health. It helps stimulate the immune system, control cell development and replication, and increase calcium absorption. While it is vital to consult your doctor before taking any new supplement, Vitamin D is regarded as a safe and effective strategy to promote urinary tract health and avoid UTIs. By taking care of your urinary system, you may preserve excellent health and lower the chance of developing major health issues.

IV. Urinary Tract Infections and Prevention

A. Understanding UTIs

Urinary tract infections, often known as UTIs, are a common condition that affects individuals of all ages, although women are more prone to this illness. UTIs are a form of bacterial infection that may arise anywhere in the urinary system, including the bladder, urethra, ureters, and kidneys.

The urinary system is made of numerous sections that work together to eliminate waste materials and excess fluid from the body. The bladder holds pee, which is ultimately released via the urethra. The ureters convey urine from the kidneys to the bladder, while the kidneys filter waste from the circulation.

When bacteria enter the urinary system and grow, it may cause an infection. The most prevalent cause of UTIs is the bacteria Escherichia coli (E. coli), which is found in the stomach and anus. UTIs may also be caused by other bacteria, such as Staphylococcus and Proteus mirabilis.

The symptoms of a UTI may vary from mild to severe, depending on the severity of the infection and where it originates in the urinary system. Some of the most frequent symptoms are a strong and persistent need to pee, a burning feeling while urinating, murky or strong-smelling urine, and pelvic discomfort. In extreme circumstances, a person may have fever, chills, and back discomfort.

Diagnosing a UTI may be done by a physical exam and a urine sample. A doctor may also do a culture test to discover the kind of bacteria causing the illness and choose the most effective therapy.

Treating a UTI includes medications to destroy the germs causing the illness. It is vital to finish the whole course of antibiotics, even if the symptoms improve, to ensure that the infection is thoroughly cured. In extreme situations, hospitalization and intravenous antibiotics may be essential.

Preventing UTIs entails taking efforts to limit the likelihood of germs entering the urinary system. Women are encouraged to wipe front to back after using the toilet, urinate before and after sexual activity, and drink lots of water. Women should also avoid using douches, powders, and other preparations in the vaginal region.

Men may also minimize their risk of UTIs by exercising excellent hygiene, wiping front to back after using the restroom, and wearing breathable underwear. Men who have had a UTI in the past or have other risk factors, such as a history of prostate issues, should take additional care to lower their risk.

In addition to lifestyle modifications, there are also additional precautions that may be done to avoid UTIs, such as taking antibiotics before and after certain operations, such as a catheterization or surgery. Women who get recurrent UTIs may benefit from taking a low-dose antibiotic daily to avoid infections.

It is vital to get medical care if you feel that you have a UTI, since untreated infections may lead to problems, such as kidney damage. Early treatment is vital to ensure that the infection is thoroughly cured and to avoid any long-term health concerns.

In conclusion, UTIs are a common sort of bacterial illness that may affect anybody, although women are more prone to this infection. UTIs may vary from moderate to severe, depending on the severity of the infection and where it occurs in the urinary system. Treatment requires medicines, and avoiding UTIs entails practicing basic hygiene and adopting lifestyle modifications. If you feel that you have a UTI, it is crucial to get medical treatment as soon as possible to avoid any long-term health concerns.

B. Risk Factors for UTIs

Urinary tract infections (UTIs) are a frequent form of infection that affect the urinary system, which includes the bladder, urethra, ureters, and kidneys. UTIs may vary from mild to severe and, if left untreated, can lead to significant problems. Understanding the risk factors for UTIs may help avoid the start of this infection.

Female anatomy: Women have a shorter urethra than males, which enables germs to more readily enter the bladder and cause an infection. Additionally, the urethra is placed near the anus, which might increase the likelihood of germs entering the urinary system.

Sexual activity: Sexual intercourse may raise the risk of UTIs because it can introduce germs into the urinary system. Women who have regular sexual intercourse or who use particular methods of birth control, such as diaphragms or spermicidal drugs, have an increased risk of UTIs.

Menopause: As women reach menopause, the normal hormonal changes that occur may lead to a fall in estrogen levels, which can raise the risk of UTIs. This is because estrogen helps to maintain the urinary system healthy and protects against bacterial infections.

Pregnancy: Pregnant women are at a greater risk of UTIs owing to the changes in the structure of the urinary system during pregnancy. Hormonal changes, greater strain on the bladder, and lower immunity may all contribute to the higher risk of UTIs during pregnancy.

Urinary catheterization: Urinary catheterization, which is a medical treatment that involves inserting a tube into the bladder to drain urine, may raise the risk of UTIs. The treatment may introduce germs into the bladder, and the extended use of a catheter can also cause damage to the bladder and urinary system, making it easier for bacteria to develop an infection.

Poor cleanliness: Poor hygiene may raise the risk of UTIs by enabling germs to enter the urinary system. Women should always wipe front to back after using the toilet, and should avoid using strong soaps or other irritants on the vaginal region.

Bladder problems: Certain medical abnormalities that affect the bladder, such as an enlarged prostate, might increase the risk of UTIs. In addition, some medical operations, such as bladder surgery, might potentially raise the risk of UTIs.

Use of certain drugs: Certain medications, such as antibiotics, might raise the risk of UTIs by killing off the healthy bacteria in the urinary system, making it easier for dangerous bacteria to create an infection. Women who use antibiotics regularly or for an extended period of time are at an increased risk of UTIs.

Weak immune system: People with compromised immune systems, such as those with HIV/AIDS or who have received an organ transplant, are at a greater risk of UTIs. This is because a weak immune system might make it more difficult for the body to fight against bacterial infections.

Family history: A family history of UTIs might raise the incidence of this illness. Women who have a mother or sister with a history of UTIs are at an increased risk of acquiring UTIs themselves.

It is crucial to understand the risk factors for UTIs in order to take efforts to avoid the start of this ailment. Some of the activities that may be done to lower the risk of UTIs include practicing excellent hygiene, drinking lots of water, peeing frequently, and avoiding the use of certain kinds of birth control. In addition, women who are at a greater risk of UTIs might consider taking antibiotics prophylactically, or utilizing a particular form of estrogen treatment to assist guard against UTIs.

C. Prevention Techniques

Urinary tract infections (UTIs) are a prevalent health condition, impacting millions of individuals every year. UTIs are caused by bacteria that enter the urinary system and grow, leading to infection and inflammation. The urinary system contains the bladder, urethra, ureters, and kidneys, and an infection may arise in any of these sites. UTIs may produce a variety of symptoms, including discomfort, burning, frequent urination, and murky urine.

While UTIs may be annoying and sometimes painful, they are typically curable with medication. However, in certain circumstances, the infection may become persistent and lead to more significant health concerns, such as kidney damage. To lower the incidence of UTIs, it is vital to maintain basic hygiene and be cognizant of lifestyle variables that might raise the risk of infection.

We will examine some of the most successful ways for avoiding and treating urinary tract infections.

Drink lots of water: Drinking enough of water is one of the greatest strategies to lower the risk of UTIs. When you drink enough water, you wash away germs and other toxins from your urinary system, minimizing the chance of illness. Aim to drink at least 8 glasses of water every day to maintain your urinary system healthy and hydrated.

Urinate often Frequent: urine is vital for avoiding UTIs because it helps clear away germs from the urinary system. If you wait too long to pee, germs may build up in the urinary system, increasing the risk of infection. Make sure to go to the restroom as soon as you feel the desire to urinate.

Practice excellent hygiene: Good cleanliness is vital for avoiding UTIs. Always wipe front to back after using the restroom to avoid germs from migrating from the anus to the urethra. Also, avoid using strong soaps or bubble baths that might irritate the sensitive tissues of the urinary system.

Wear breathable underwear: Wearing breathable underwear may help lower the incidence of UTIs by keeping the region surrounding the urethra dry and minimizing the possibility of bacteria development. Opt for cotton underwear or cotton-lined pantyhose to keep the region surrounding the urethra dry and pleasant.

Avoid holding in urine: Holding in urine for lengthy periods of time may raise the risk of UTIs by enabling bacteria to proliferate in the urinary system. If you need to go to the restroom, go as soon as possible.

Avoid using feminine hygiene products: Feminine hygiene products, such as douches and powders, may irritate the sensitive tissues of the urinary system, increasing the risk of UTIs. If you are prone to UTIs, stop taking these items or speak to your doctor about alternate choices.

Take antibiotics as indicated If you are diagnosed with a UTI, your doctor will likely prescribe medications to treat the infection. It is vital to take the antibiotics as advised and to finish the whole course of therapy, even if your symptoms have improved. Failure to finish the whole course of antibiotics may lead to antibiotic resistance, making it more difficult to treat subsequent UTIs.

Use a heating pad: Applying a heating pad to the lower belly might help ease the pain and discomfort associated with UTIs. The warmth of the heating pad may assist enhance blood flow and decrease inflammation, speeding up the healing process.

Try over-the-counter pain medications: Over-the-counter pain medications, such as ibuprofen or acetaminophen, may help reduce the pain and discomfort associated with UTIs. However, it is crucial to consult your doctor before taking any new drug.

D. Antibiotics and Alternative Treatments

Urinary tract infections (UTIs) are one of the most frequent forms of diseases, impacting millions of individuals each year. UTIs are caused by bacteria that enter the urinary system and produce symptoms such as discomfort, burning during urination, frequent urination, and murky or strong-smelling urine. In extreme situations, a UTI may lead to kidney damage, and in rare circumstances, sepsis (a life-threatening infection that spreads throughout the body) (a life-threatening infection that spreads throughout the body). Antibiotics are the most frequent therapy for UTIs, however with the growth of antibiotic resistance, other therapies are becoming more popular.

Antibiotics are the main therapy for UTIs. They operate by destroying the microorganisms that cause the ailment. Antibiotics are normally recommended for three to seven days, and patients are urged to take the whole course of antibiotics, even if they start to feel better before the course is complete. This is because the antibiotics need to be taken long enough to kill all of the germs, otherwise the bacteria may grow resistant to the medicines and the illness may recur.

Common antibiotics used to treat UTIs include amoxicillin, ciprofloxacin, and nitrofurantoin. While antibiotics are very successful in treating UTIs, they also have significant disadvantages. Antibiotics may produce side effects, such as nausea, diarrhea, and allergic reactions. Additionally, abuse of antibiotics has led to a rise in antibiotic resistance. This implies that germs are developing resistance to antibiotics, making it more difficult to treat illnesses.

In light of these concerns, more individuals are turning to alternative therapies for UTIs. Some of the most common alternative therapies include herbal medicines, probiotics, and lifestyle adjustments.

Herbal remedies are natural medicines that are used to cure a range of health ailments. Some of the most often utilized herbs for UTIs are cranberry, uva , and goldenrod. Cranberry has been demonstrated to inhibit bacteria from sticking to the urinary system, while uva ursi may aid to decrease inflammation and improve symptoms of UTIs. Goldenrod is another popular herb for UTIs, and it has been proven to have antiseptic and diuretic characteristics, which may help to flush out germs and lessen the incidence of UTIs.

Probiotics are living microorganisms that are helpful to the gut. Probiotics may assist to restore the balance of healthy bacteria in the stomach, which helps prevent UTIs from forming. Some of the most often utilized probiotics for UTIs are Lactobacillus and Bifidobacterium. These probiotics are present in many fermented foods, such as yogurt, kefir, and sauerkraut. They may also be taken in supplement form.

Lifestyle modifications may also play a role in preventing and treating UTIs. Drinking enough water may assist to flush out germs from the urinary system, and avoiding tight clothes can minimize the incidence of UTIs by enabling good ventilation and minimizing moisture. Wiping from front to back after using the bathroom may also help to lower the incidence of UTIs, since this stops germs from moving from the anus to the urethra.

In conclusion, UTIs are a prevalent and unpleasant infection that affects millions of individuals each year. Antibiotics are the main therapy for UTIs, however with the growth of antibiotic resistance, other therapies are becoming more popular. Some of the most common alternative therapies include herbal medicines, probiotics, and lifestyle adjustments. While antibiotics are very effective, they also have certain downsides, such as side effects and the potential of antibiotic resistance. By adopting alternative remedies into their healthcare practice, individuals may lower the risk of UTIs and enhance their general health and well-being.

V. Bladder Health and Incontinence

A. Understanding Bladder Health

Bladder health is a vital element of general health and well-being, although it is frequently disregarded or not spoken about as freely as other health problems. Understanding bladder health entails being aware of the architecture of the bladder, typical bladder disorders, and the measures you can take to maintain excellent bladder health.

The bladder is a muscular sac found in the pelvis that holds urine generated by the kidneys. When the bladder is full, messages are delivered to the brain to let you know it's time to pee. As the bladder muscles contract, urine is evacuated from the body via the urethra. The bladder and the muscles that govern its function are part of the lower urinary tract system.

Common bladder disorders might include urinary incontinence (leaking pee), urinary urgency (a sudden, urgent desire to urinate), urinary frequency (needing to urinate often), and painful urination (dysuria) (dysuria). Some bladder disorders are brief and readily managed, while others may be an indication of a more severe underlying illness.

Urinary incontinence may be caused by several circumstances, including weak bladder muscles, nerve injury, or difficulties with the pelvic floor muscles. In women, childbearing and menopause may also lead to incontinence.

Urinary urgency and frequency may be indications of an overactive bladder, which is a disease in which the bladder muscle spasms suddenly, prompting an urgent desire to pee. This may be caused by nerve injury, bladder muscle difficulties, or an enlarged prostate in males.

Painful urination may be caused by bladder or urinary tract infections, bladder stones, or an inflammation of the bladder. In certain situations, painful urination may also be an indication of a more severe ailment such as bladder cancer.

To maintain healthy bladder health, it is vital to exercise excellent bladder practices. This includes:

Drinking enough of water: Staying hydrated is crucial for general health and may help wash away germs from the urinary system, lowering the chance of infection.

Timing your fluid intake: Avoid drinking big quantities of fluid in the evening, since this might lead to repeated visits to the toilet throughout the night.

Regular toilet breaks: Regular bathroom breaks may help train the bladder and avoid urine incontinence.

Pelvic floor exercises: Strengthening the pelvic floor muscles may assist improve bladder control and minimize the chance of incontinence.

Avoiding bladder irritants: Certain foods and beverages, such as coffee, alcohol, and spicy meals, may irritate the bladder and increase symptoms of bladder disorders.

Quitting smoking: Smoking may raise the risk of bladder cancer and can also aggravate bladder disorders such as incontinence.

Maintaining a healthy weight: Being overweight or obese may place additional strain on the bladder and increase the risk of incontinence.

It is also crucial to get medical assistance if you develop any chronic bladder issues. Your doctor can assist determine the source of your symptoms and establish a treatment plan that is suited for you. Treatment options might vary from lifestyle modifications and pelvic floor exercises to drugs and surgery, depending on the origin of your symptoms.

In conclusion, bladder health is a critical part of overall health and well-being. Understanding the architecture of the bladder, typical bladder disorders, and the measures you can take to maintain excellent bladder health may help avoid bladder problems and enhance quality of life. If you encounter recurrent bladder difficulties, obtaining medical care is vital in order to receive a thorough diagnosis and successful treatment.

B. Causes of Incontinence

Incontinence is a medical disorder that affects millions of individuals worldwide, resulting in the loss of bladder or bowel control. It is a frequent condition that may greatly influence a person's quality of life, causing physical, mental, and social discomfort. In this essay, we will dig into the numerous reasons for incontinence, including both physical and psychological issues.

Physical Causes of Incontinence

Urinary Tract Infections (UTIs) - UTIs are a prevalent cause of incontinence in women. These infections may cause inflammation and edema in the bladder, making it difficult to contain pee. UTIs may also induce an overactive bladder, leading to frequent, urgent urinating.

Weak Bladder Muscles - As we age, our bladder muscles may lose their strength and suppleness, making it more tough to regulate urine. This form of incontinence is known as stress incontinence and is commonly caused by weak pelvic floor muscles.

Neurological Conditions - Certain neurological disorders, such as multiple sclerosis, Parkinson's disease, and spinal cord injuries, may influence the nerve impulses that govern bladder function, resulting in incontinence.

Prostate Problems - Men might also develop incontinence as a consequence of an enlarged prostate or prostate cancer. These disorders may exert pressure on the urethra and bladder, making it difficult to contain pee.

Childbirth - Women who have given birth may develop incontinence owing to straining and injury to the pelvic floor muscles during delivery. This form of incontinence is termed stress incontinence and may result in the flow of urine during physical exercise or even laughing.

Psychological Causes of Incontinence

Anxiety and Stress - People who suffer from anxiety and stress may develop incontinence owing to the psychological influence these illnesses have on the body. When we encounter worry or stress, our bodies go into "fight or flight" mode, resulting in increased muscular tension and impaired bladder control.

Depression - Depression may also contribute to incontinence, since it typically leads to a diminished sensation of control over one's own body. This might result in an overactive bladder, producing frequent and urgent urinating.

Psychological Trauma - Individuals who have undergone psychological trauma, such as sexual assault or a traumatic incident, may also develop incontinence as a consequence of the psychological effect of the trauma.

Dementia and Alzheimer's Disease - People with dementia and Alzheimer's disease may develop incontinence as a consequence of the cognitive deterioration that happens with these disorders. They may forget to use the restroom, or have difficulties finding their way to the bathroom.

In conclusion, incontinence is a complicated medical problem that may be caused by a range of physical and psychological reasons. Understanding the fundamental cause of incontinence is vital in designing successful treatment regimens and improving the quality of life for people afflicted. Whether it is due to weak bladder muscles, neurological abnormalities, psychological trauma, or any other underlying reason, it is vital to seek the advice of a healthcare expert to treat this issue. With adequate medical treatment and support, people may reclaim control over their bodies and enjoy a greater quality of life.

C. Treatment Options

Bladder health and incontinence are significant problems for individuals of all ages. Incontinence refers to the lack of control over urine, which may be caused by different underlying disorders. The good news is that there are a range of treatment options available for bladder health and incontinence, ranging from lifestyle modifications to drugs and surgery. In this post, we will discuss the numerous therapies available to help you recover control over your bladder and enhance your quality of life.

Lifestyle Changes

One of the easiest and most efficient therapies for incontinence is to adopt specific lifestyle adjustments. This might involve basic modifications such as reducing your fluid consumption, avoiding bladder irritants like coffee and alcohol, and lowering weight if you are overweight. Additionally, exercising pelvic floor exercises, often known as Kegels, may help strengthen the muscles that govern urine.

Bladder Training

Bladder training is another non-invasive therapy method that may be useful for persons with incontinence. This entails gradually extending the duration between toilet visits, helping to retrain the bladder to retain more pee for longer periods of time. This therapy is commonly used in combination with pelvic floor exercises and is especially useful for patients with urge incontinence.

Medications

There are a range of drugs available to address incontinence, including antimuscarinics, beta-3 agonists, and tricyclic antidepressants. Antimuscarinics operate by relaxing the bladder muscles and lowering urine urgency and frequency. Beta-3 agonists are a newer kind of drug that function by stimulating the bladder muscles and increasing bladder control. Tricyclic antidepressants may be useful for persons with stress incontinence since they assist to strengthen the strength of the pelvic floor muscles.

Surgery

In more extreme situations, surgery may be required to address incontinence. The most prevalent surgical techniques are sling operations, bladder suspension procedures, and bulking agents. Sling treatments entail putting a sling over the bladder neck to support the urethra and avoid incontinence. Bladder suspension methods entail raising and repositioning the bladder to restore normal function. Bulking drugs are injected into the tissues surrounding the urethra to aid enhance bladder control.

Pelvic Floor Physical Therapy

Pelvic floor physical therapy is another treatment option that may be useful for persons with incontinence. This sort of treatment works on the muscles, nerves, and connective tissue in the pelvis and may help to improve bladder control and minimize urine incontinence. Physical therapy may also assist to relieve pelvic discomfort, enhance sexual function, and treat other associated disorders.

Botox Injections

Botox injections are a relatively recent therapy option for incontinence and have been demonstrated to be useful for patients with overactive bladder syndrome. Botox works by relaxing the muscles in the bladder, lowering urine urgency and frequency, and increasing bladder control. This therapy is normally conducted as an outpatient procedure and typically takes less than an hour to complete.

In conclusion, there are a range of therapies available for bladder health and incontinence, including lifestyle modifications, bladder training, drugs, surgery, pelvic floor physical therapy, and Botox injections. The optimal treatment choice for you will depend on the underlying cause of your incontinence and the severity of your symptoms. It is vital to chat with your healthcare practitioner to identify the best course of therapy for your unique requirements. With the correct therapy, you may recover control over your bladder and enhance your quality of life.

D. Pelvic Floor Exercises for Improved Bladder Control

Pelvic floor exercises are vital for improving bladder control in both men and women. These workouts may be done anywhere, at any time, and without any equipment. They are meant to strengthen the muscles in the pelvic area, which may help avoid urine incontinence and enhance bladder control. In this post, we will cover the necessity of pelvic floor exercises and how to practice them effectively for optimal results.

Urinary incontinence is a widespread issue that affects millions of individuals worldwide. It happens when the muscles in the pelvic area are weak, which may lead to involuntary pee leaking. Women are more prone to urine incontinence than males, particularly after pregnancy and delivery. However, anybody might encounter bladder control challenges owing to age, weight, or certain medical disorders.

The pelvic floor muscles are crucial for supporting the bladder, uterus, and rectum. These muscles assist regulate the discharge of urine and feces, and they play a key function in maintaining bladder control. If the pelvic floor muscles are weak, they can't offer the essential support, resulting in urine incontinence.

Pelvic floor exercises may help strengthen these muscles, reducing urine incontinence and increasing bladder control. These exercises are also known as Kegels, after the doctor who invented them in the 1940s. They may be done in any posture, whether you are seated, standing, or laying down.

To execute pelvic floor exercises, you need to start by locating the proper muscles. The best approach to achieve this is by attempting to interrupt the flow of pee mid-stream. The muscles you employ to achieve this are called the pelvic floor muscles. Once you have identified these muscles, you may start practicing pelvic floor exercises.

There are various techniques to practice pelvic floor exercises, including:

Slow contractions: In this exercise, you slowly contract the pelvic floor muscles and hold for 5 to 10 seconds. Then, gently release and rest for 5 to 10 seconds. Repeat this exercise 10 to 15 times.

Quick contractions: In this exercise, you swiftly contract and release the pelvic floor muscles repeatedly. Try to accomplish 10 to 20 repetitions in a row.

Long contractions: In this exercise, you tighten the pelvic floor muscles and hold for 10 to 20 seconds. Then, rest for 10 to 20 seconds. Repeat this exercise 5 to 10 times.

Combination contractions: In this workout, you complete a moderate contraction followed by a fast contraction, and then a gradual release. Repeat this process 10 to 15 times.

It's vital to practice these exercises properly to minimize injury and gain maximum benefits. When conducting pelvic floor exercises, be sure to:

Breathe normally: Avoid holding your breath throughout the workouts. Instead, concentrate on breathing regularly as you contract and relax the pelvic floor muscles.

Isolate the pelvic floor muscles: Make sure you just engage the pelvic floor muscles and avoid contracting other muscles, such as the abdomen, legs, or butt.

Focus on form: Pay attention to the technique, making sure to tense and release the muscles appropriately.

Progressively raise the intensity: Start with a few repetitions and gradually increase the number of repetitions as you grow stronger.

Conduct routinely: It's crucial to perform pelvic floor exercises regularly to gain optimal results. Aim to complete these exercises at least three times a day.

Pelvic floor exercises may be done anywhere, at any time, and without any equipment. This makes them a fantastic alternative for anybody trying to enhance bladder control, whether at home, work, or on the road.

VI. Menopause and Urinary Tract Health

A. Understanding Menopause and Its Effects

Menopause is a normal biological process that signals the end of a woman's reproductive years. It happens when the ovaries cease releasing eggs, and the levels of hormones, such as estrogen and progesterone, decline drastically. This may lead to a variety of physical, emotional, and psychological changes. Understanding menopause and its impacts is vital for women reaching this point in their life, as well as for the people around them who wish to assist them.

The onset of menopause is varied for every woman, with some experiencing it as early as their mid-30s, while others may not reach it until their late 50s. The average age of menopause is 51 years old, and it is considered to be complete if a woman has gone 12 consecutive months without a menstrual cycle. However, some women may have perimenopause, which is the transition phase preceding menopause, for many years prior to the start of menopause.

One of the most well-known consequences of menopause is hot flashes, which are characterized by a sudden sense of heat and perspiration, typically accompanied by a fast pulse. They may be fairly severe and last anywhere from a few seconds to many minutes. Other frequent symptoms of menopause include night sweats, vaginal dryness, sleep difficulties, mood fluctuations, and diminished libido. Some women may also report joint discomfort, memory lapses, and difficulties focusing.

In addition to these physical symptoms, menopause may also have a substantial influence on a woman's emotional and psychological well-being. Many women report feeling worried, angry, and even melancholy during this period. Some may suffer sentiments of grief and loss, since the end of their reproductive years might bring up thoughts of aging and death. For some women, these emotional shifts may be extremely tough, since they may feel like they are losing a part of themselves.

It is crucial to remember that these symptoms are typical and that many women experience them throughout menopause. It is particularly vital to seek medical assistance if these symptoms grow severe or interfere with everyday living. Hormonal replacement therapy (HRT) may be a helpful treatment for certain women, and it includes taking estrogen and progesterone to help balance the levels of hormones in the body. However, it is crucial to explore the risks and advantages of HRT with a healthcare physician before commencing any medication.

In addition to medical therapy, there are various lifestyle adjustments that may help women manage the symptoms of menopause. Exercise is one of the most effective strategies to manage hot flashes, since it helps regulate body temperature and lower stress levels. Eating a nutritious diet and avoiding triggers, such as coffee and alcohol, may also help lessen hot flashes and other symptoms. Maintaining appropriate sleep patterns is also crucial, as it may help decrease tiredness and enhance mood.

One of the most essential things women may do throughout menopause is to seek assistance from loved ones and healthcare experts. Talking to a trusted friend or family member about the problems of menopause may be immensely beneficial, and seeking the assistance of a healthcare practitioner can help women manage their symptoms and navigate this period in their life. There are also support groups for women going through menopause, which may provide a safe and encouraging place for women to discuss their experiences and give each other advice and support.

In conclusion, menopause is a normal biological process that signals the end of a woman's reproductive years and may lead to a variety of physical, emotional, and psychological changes. Understanding these changes and receiving assistance may help women manage the symptoms of menopause and navigate this period in their life with confidence.

B. Urinary Tract Changes During Menopause

Menopause is a period in a woman's life when the ovaries cease releasing eggs and the production of hormones such as estrogen and progesterone declines. This stage is defined by a multitude of physical and emotional changes, including alterations in the urinary tract. The urinary tract is a system of organs that comprises the bladder, urethra, and kidneys, which work together to generate, store, and remove urine from the body. During menopause, the urinary system is influenced by hormonal changes, which may produce a multitude of symptoms that can vary from moderate to severe. In this post, we will explore the urinary tract alterations that occur during menopause, what causes these changes, and how they might be controlled.

One of the most prevalent urinary tract alterations after menopause is urine incontinence. Urinary incontinence is the lack of bladder control, which may result in inadvertent leaks or accidents. This illness is caused by the reduction in estrogen levels after menopause, which may weaken the muscles that support the bladder. The drop in estrogen levels also affects the urethral sphincter, which is responsible for keeping urine from seeping out of the bladder. As a consequence, women who develop urine incontinence after menopause may encounter unintended leaks when they cough, sneeze, laugh, or participate in physical exercise.

Another typical urinary tract alteration after menopause is urine frequency. This ailment is defined by the need to pee more regularly than normal, and may vary from going to the toilet every hour to wanting to urinate multiple times throughout the night. Urinary frequency is caused by the fall in estrogen levels, which may lead the bladder to become less elastic, making it harder for it to store more pee. Women who have urinary frequency during menopause may also experience urgent urination, which is the sudden and acute desire to pee.

Urinary tract infections (UTIs) are another prevalent alteration following menopause. UTIs are caused by bacteria that enter the urinary system and affect the bladder, urethra, or kidneys. During menopause, the fall in estrogen levels might produce changes in the urinary system that make it more sensitive to UTIs. For example, estrogen helps to maintain the bladder and urethral walls healthy, but when estrogen levels fall, the walls of the bladder and urethra may become thin and inflamed, making it easier for germs to infect the urinary system.

Vaginal dryness is another urinary tract alteration that may develop after menopause. Vaginal dryness is caused by the drop in estrogen levels, which may cause the vaginal walls to become thin and less moisturized. This disease may make sexual intercourse painful and can also raise the risk of UTIs. The drop in estrogen levels may also cause the urethral sphincter to weaken, making it harder to regulate the flow of pee, which can lead to urinary incontinence.

In addition to these urinary tract alterations, women who undergo menopause may also have changes in their menstrual cycles. The menstrual cycle is governed by hormones like estrogen and progesterone, and when these chemicals diminish throughout menopause, the menstrual cycle may become irregular, leading to a variety of symptoms, including hot flashes, night sweats, and vaginal dryness.

Managing urinary tract changes throughout menopause may be a struggle, but there are a variety of medications available to assist women manage these symptoms. For example, pelvic floor muscle exercises may assist to strengthen the muscles that support the bladder, which can help to lower the risk of urine incontinence. Drinking enough of water may also assist to wash out germs from the urinary system and minimize the risk of UTIs.

C. Treatment Options for Menopausal Urinary Tract Issues

Menopause is a normal period in a woman's life that generally happens between the ages of 45 and 55. During this period, the body experiences a drop in hormones, particularly estrogen, which may contribute to a range of symptoms such as hot flashes, nocturnal sweats, and mood changes. One of the most frequent, but often neglected, symptoms of menopause is urinary tract difficulties.

Urinary tract troubles during menopause are frequently caused by the weakening of the tissues in the urethra, which may result in impaired bladder control, urgency, and frequency of urine. The good news is that there are various effective therapeutic options available to assist control these symptoms.

One of the most prevalent treatments for urinary tract difficulties after menopause is hormone therapy (HT) (HT). HT entails taking estrogen or a mixture of estrogen and progesterone to help balance hormones in the body and give relief from symptoms like vaginal dryness and hot flashes. HT is available in numerous forms, including oral tablets, lotions, and patches.

HT may also be used to assist address urinary tract disorders. This is because estrogen plays a critical function in maintaining the health of the bladder and urethra. The higher amounts of estrogen from hormone treatment may help strengthen the tissues in these locations and improve bladder control. However, it is crucial to remember that hormone treatment does come with its own set of hazards, so it is vital to consult with a healthcare expert to establish whether it is the appropriate choice for you.

In addition to hormone medication, pelvic floor exercises may also be a beneficial technique in controlling urinary tract difficulties. These exercises include strengthening the muscles in the pelvic region, including the bladder and urethra, to enhance bladder control and minimize symptoms such as urgency and frequency of urinating.

There are various different forms of pelvic floor exercises, including Kegel exercises and biofeedback, so it is vital to engage with a healthcare practitioner to decide the best course of action for you.

Another method for addressing urinary tract difficulties during menopause is bladder training. This includes gradually extending the length of time between visits to the toilet to assist improve bladder capacity and decrease the frequency of urine. Bladder training may also assist with other symptoms, such as urgency and midnight urination.

Medications may also be a valuable aid in controlling urinary tract difficulties during menopause. Anticholinergic medicines may be used to assist relax the bladder and lessen symptoms such as urgency and frequency. Other drugs, including estrogen creams and pessaries, may be used to assist treat vaginal dryness and enhance bladder function.

Surgery is another option for addressing urinary tract difficulties during menopause. This may be advised for women with severe urine incontinence or other urinary tract disorders that do not respond to other kinds of therapy. Some typical forms of surgery include slings, bladder neck suspensions, and urethral bulking agents.

In conclusion, urinary tract disorders during menopause may be an unpleasant and painful experience, but they are controllable. Whether it's via hormone therapy, pelvic floor exercises, bladder training, drugs, or surgery, there are various effective treatment options available to assist control these symptoms. It is vital to consult with a healthcare practitioner to identify the best course of action for you and to ensure that you get the most suitable and successful therapy. With the correct care and attention, it is possible to overcome these symptoms and lead a healthy and meaningful life throughout menopause.

VII. Conclusion

Empowering women to take charge of their urinary tract health is vital in ensuring they experience a healthy and meaningful life. Urinary tract health influences various elements of a woman's life, including her physical, emotional, and mental well-being. Despite this, many women are not well educated about their urinary tract health, and frequently suffer in silence owing to the shame associated with talking about this condition. The objective of this article is to educate and empower women to take care of their urinary tract health and to give them the tools and information they need to avoid and manage common urinary tract disorders.

The urinary tract is a complicated system that begins at the kidneys and terminates at the urethra. It is responsible for eliminating waste and surplus water from the body, which is ultimately expelled as urine. A healthy urinary system is vital for maintaining overall health and wellbeing, but when it is not operating correctly, it may lead to a variety of issues, including urinary incontinence, urinary tract infections, and bladder disorders.

Urinary incontinence is a widespread condition impacting millions of women globally. It is the involuntary loss of urine and may be caused by a number of causes, including pregnancy, menopause, and certain medical problems. While it is a curable ailment, many women suffer in silence, feeling humiliated and ashamed to address it with their healthcare professional. The good news is that there are a number of therapies available, including pelvic floor exercises, bladder training, and medication, which may help women recover control of their bladder and improve their quality of life.

Urinary tract infections (UTIs) are another major concern affecting women. UTIs are caused by bacteria that enter the urinary system and grow, creating an infection. UTIs may produce a number of symptoms, including painful urination, frequent urination, and a strong need to pee. While UTIs are not always avoidable, there are precautions women may do to lower their risk, including wiping front to back after using the bathroom, wearing breathable underwear, and drinking lots of water. If a woman feels she has a UTI, it is crucial that she receives medical assistance as quickly as possible, since UTIs may lead to significant problems if left untreated.